D0926840

Everything
You Need to
Know About

Human
Papillomavirus

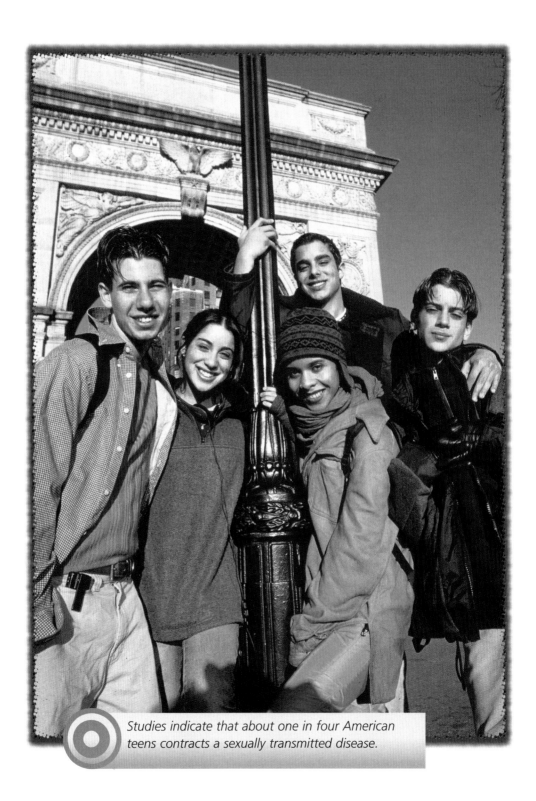

Studies indicate that about one in four American teens contracts a sexually transmitted disease.

Everything You Need to Know About
Human Papillomavirus

Elizabeth Carter

The Rosen Publishing Group, Inc.
New York

The author wishes to thank Suzanne Holm, M.S., A.R.N.P., for her help in understanding and describing the anatomy of the cervix and the transformational zone. Additional assistance was provided by the National STD and AIDS Prevention Hotline, the American Cancer Society, and the American Social Health Association's HPV and Cervical Cancer Prevention Resource Center.

Published in 2001 by The Rosen Publishing Group, Inc.
29 East 21st Street, New York, NY 10010

First Edition

Library of Congress Cataloging-in-Publication Data

Carter, Elizabeth, 1959–
Everything you need to know about human papillomavirus / by Elizabeth Carter.—1st ed.
p. cm. — (The need to know library)
Includes bibliographical references and index.
ISBN 0-8239-3397-0 (library binding)
1. Papillomavirus diseases—Juvenile literature. [1. Papillomavirus diseases. 2. Diseases.]
[DNLM: 1. Papillomavirus, Human—pathogenicity—Popular Works. 2. Papovaviridae Infections—Popular Works. 3. Tumor Virus Infections—Popular Works. WC 500 C323e 2001] I. Title. II. Series.
RC168.P15 C37 2001
616'.0194—dc21

00-012609

Manufactured in the United States of America

Contents

Introduction

Every year in the United States, three million teenagers contract some type of sexually transmitted disease, or STD. While most think it will never happen to them, studies from the Alan Guttmacher Institute and the Kaiser Family Foundation reveal that about one in four American teens becomes infected.

According to the American Social Health Association, the most common STD in the United States today is a group of viruses known as human papillomavirus, or HPV. A virus is made up of protein and genetic material (DNA) that is capable of cell growth and multiplication within the body or host that it invades. While most of these HPV viruses are considered harmless, some cause genital warts. Scientists now know that it is more common for people to develop HPV without symptoms than it is for them to exhibit signs of genital warts. These HPV infections are classified as low-risk infections. Other higher-risk strains (similar types) of HPV (strains 16, 18, 31, 33, and 45) are linked to certain cancers in women and others in men, but are not likely to cause genital warts. Fortunately, changes in technology and advancements in research have armed doctors with more information about cancer-causing HPV strains.

An article in the February 28, 2000, issue of *American Medical News* puts the number of new HPV infections in the United States at an estimated five and a half million each year. HPV has become so widespread that as many as 20 million people are believed to have an active genital HPV infection at any point in time, a fact confirmed by the Guttmacher Institute and other experts.

HPV isn't just an American problem either. The January 2000 issue of *Chatelaine*, a Canadian magazine, reported that between 40 and 80 percent of Canadian women of childbearing age have contracted an HPV infection. HPV is also a worldwide problem.

If you've never heard of HPV before, you're not alone. The American Social Health Association's background report on HPV pointed out that in one national survey, 76 percent of the women respondents were completely unaware of HPV.

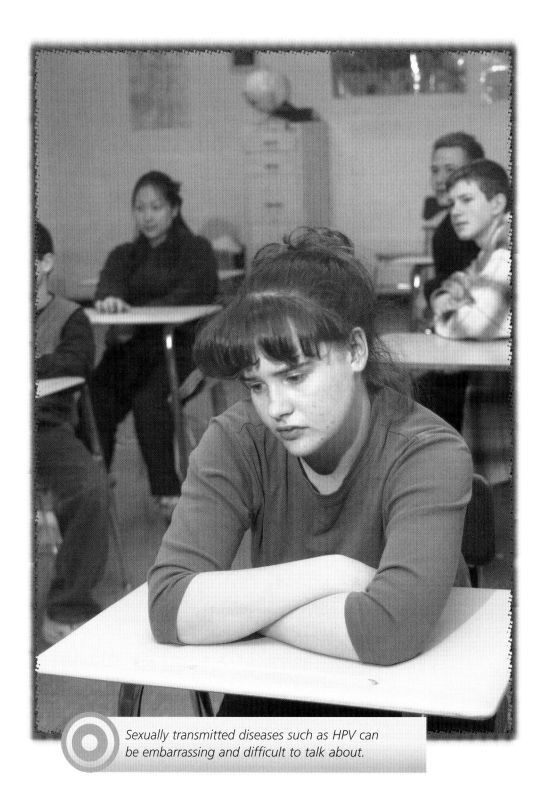

Sexually transmitted diseases such as HPV can be embarrassing and difficult to talk about.

If you are a teenager and are reading about HPV for the first time, you may rightly wonder what this means to you, where you can go for more information, and what steps you can take to protect your health.

This book will discuss HPV, its impact on the body and health of teens and adults, its symptoms, how it is spread, how it is treated, and how to minimize your exposure. HPV and genital warts, and the relationship between HPV and cancer will also be covered. Finally, sources of information and STD resources are provided.

STDs such as HPV are sometimes difficult to talk about. Teens are often embarrassed because of the stigma associated with STDs. It is very important to address this subject since many STDs, including HPV, have no obvious symptoms because the body's immune system fights these diseases while they are developing. If you are not aware of the facts, it is often difficult to tell if you're in need of treatment or if you have been infected. This is one reason HPV and other STDs are so easily spread; some people don't even know that they are infected and are infecting others.

Reading this book is a valuable first step toward overcoming any awkwardness you may feel about STDs. It will also help you make responsible decisions about your health and sexual behavior.

Chapter 1

What Is HPV?

Human papillomavirus, or HPV, causes an infection that one person can give to another during sex or pre-sexual activities. HPV refers to a group of more than eighty viruses and is one of the most common STDs in both men and women. HPV is sometimes referred to as the "wart virus" because it is most often associated with the warts that some strains of HPV can cause on the genitals as well as those found on other parts of the body, such as the hands and feet.

Some of the strains of HPV that we will concern ourselves with in this book can lead to the development of certain types of cancer. HPV is now known to be the leading cause of cancer of the cervix (the portion of the uterus that opens into the vagina) in women. Known as genital warts, or venereal warts, these growths, in addition to appearing on all parts of the genitals, can grow on, in, or around the anus and inside the vagina. Genital

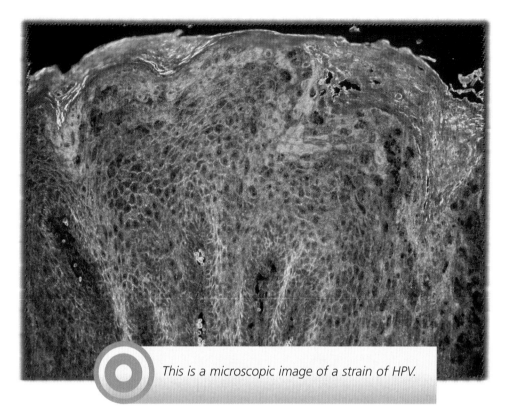

warts may also appear on the outer pubic skin, the groin area, and the areas near the inner thigh.

In some cases, genital warts can become quite large and grow to resemble cauliflower. However, they may be overlooked if they are small, flat, flesh-colored, or painless. Symptoms such as itching, bleeding, or pain are not common but can occur. Or, you may be infected with HPV and show no symptoms at all.

The strains of lower-risk HPV that lead to genital warts are distinct from those that produce warts on the hands and feet. These also vary from the more serious high-risk types of HPV responsible for cancer of the cervix in women and cancer of the penis or anus in men.

Although genital warts are an obvious sign of HPV infection, many who contract HPV never develop genital warts. In fact, most people who become infected with HPV don't even know they have it. This is because the body's immune system holds HPV at bay, leaving no visible symptoms, even though the infection is still present within the body. This means that although you have no visible symptoms, you could still infect others with HPV.

What Are Warts?

A wart is a rough, round, or oval, raised overgrowth of skin caused by HPV, an infection in the top layer of the skin. There are several types of warts. Each has a different appearance, depending on where it grows.

Warts have an interesting history and have been written about for centuries. Known to the Romans as "verrucas," genital warts were suspected to be sexually transmitted as far back as AD 25. The suggestion that warts were caused by a virus came much later, in nineteenth century England. It was only after 1950, however, when papillomavirus particles were finally analyzed under a microscope, that scientists accepted the virus connection. We now know of, and have isolated, every variety of wart, both genital (venereal) and common.

HPV thrives in the cells of the skin. Because of this, HPV can be spread through contact with infected pubic skin or other areas that condoms don't cover. Condoms

◎ Plantar warts: These are commonplace warts that appear on the soles of the feet and are sometimes dotted with tiny black or red dots, which are clotted blood vessels. When plantar warts grow in a cluster they are known as mosaic warts.

◎ Flat warts: These warts are also commonplace and appear on the face, neck, forearms, hands, or fingers and are flesh-colored, small, and flat. Flat warts tend to grow in large numbers, between twenty to one hundred at a time.

◎ Common warts (also called seed warts, periungual warts, or subungual warts): Like the name suggests, these small warts appear to be ordinary and often show up under the fingernails or toenails, or on the hands, arms, and legs, especially in children.

◎ Genital (or venereal) warts: These warts are highly contagious and spread by skin-to-skin contact, and are normally raised, fleshy growths found in the genital or anal area. This type of wart is the main subject matter of this book.

provide limited protection and should be used, but wearing a condom during sex is not a total safeguard against HPV. Condoms do, however, offer an effective barrier against other STDs and pregnancy.

The presence of HPV in the skin may result in cell changes that can be seen only with the use of a high-powered lens. HPV can also live in the skin without causing any cell alteration at all. These two factors make it hard to know when you've been infected.

Because of this, HPV has become so common that the American Social Health Association (ASHA) estimates that 80 percent of sexually active people have an active HPV infection at some point.

Many people still remain confused about HPV, how it is contracted, how it is spread, and how it develops in the body. In an effort to share accurate information with the public, health care providers, and others, the ASHA has recently set up the National HPV and Cervical Cancer Prevention Resource Center, which has a toll-free HPV hotline. In addition to the most up-to-date information on HPV and cancer prevention, the center also provides lists of community resources and support groups for those dealing with the emotional issues that follow the discovery of genital HPV or cancer. See the national HPV hotline number and other valuable information in the Where to Go for Help section in the back of this book.

Chapter 2

The Symptoms and Diagnosis of HPV and Genital Warts

Genital warts and other strains of HPV are spread through skin-to-skin contact during anal, oral, or vaginal sex with an infected person. HPV and genital warts can infect any sexually active teenager or adult. You can have sex with someone and not know that you've become infected with HPV or genital warts. This is because genital warts don't always appear quickly; in some instances, people infected with HPV don't develop any symptoms at all. HPV can live in the skin and body without any warts or changes occurring. This is called latent (unseen) HPV. You can still infect others with HPV and genital warts when you have no symptoms.

In other cases, symptoms may occur weeks, months, or years after becoming infected. Usually, however, genital warts develop between three and eight months after exposure.

Once a person is infected, HPV could lead to the following results:

◎ **Latent or inactive infection:** Infected areas appear to be normal because the body's immune system is controlling the virus. Even though you can't see any changes, you may still infect others during vaginal, oral, or anal sex.

◎ **Subclinical or active infection I:** HPV begins to cause cellular changes inside the body, which in women are sometimes seen as "abnormal" results on a Pap smear. (A Pap smear is a quick, painless test that allows doctors to collect a very small tissue sample from a woman's cervix.) These abnormal cellular changes sometimes lead to the development of cancer in both men and women.

◎ **Clinical or active infection II:** HPV begins to cause visible changes on the outside of the body in the form of genital warts. Genital warts do not lead to cancer, but their presence should alert both you and your doctor to do further testing to determine if cancer is present in the body.

Symptoms of Genital Warts

Genital (venereal) warts can appear on the outside of the penis, vulva, or opening of the anus. They may also develop inside the vagina, throat, or anus. They may be small or large, flat or raised, single or in clusters resembling cauliflower. They may also be in more than one area of the body and often develop on pubic skin, an area that condoms don't cover. This is why it is important to look at your own body, as well as your partner's, before becoming intimate. For both teens and adults, speaking frankly, openly, and honestly about STDs and their prevention is a responsible prerequisite to any sexual activity.

Any unusual growths or changes on your skin or the skin of anyone you've had sex with should be examined by a doctor, especially if you suspect you've been infected with genital warts or any other STD.

While genital warts are not life threatening, their discovery can be very frightening. It is common to feel angry with the person who you believe infected you. You may feel alone or ashamed. Remember, genital warts can be successfully treated, while helping to control their transmission to others.

Diagnosing Genital Warts

A special magnifying lens called a colposcope may be used by a doctor or nurse to clearly see warts in the

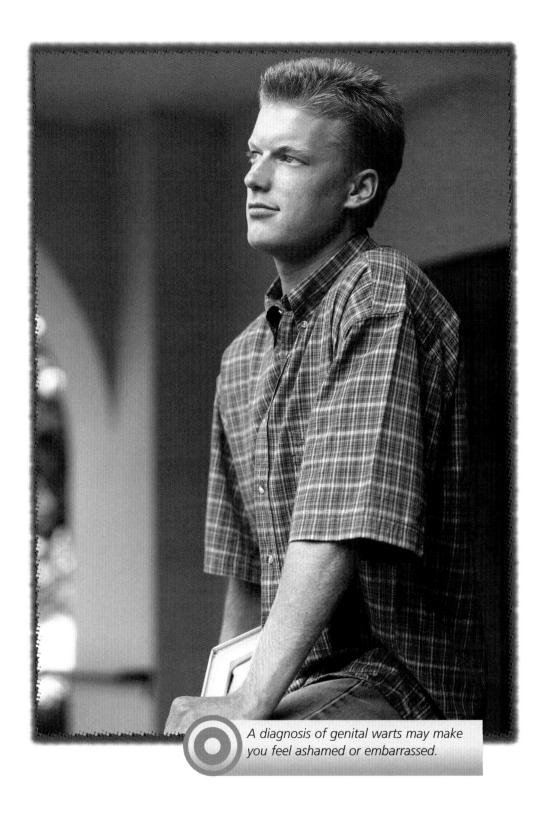

A diagnosis of genital warts may make you feel ashamed or embarrassed.

cervix or other places inside the body. This test is called a colposcopy. Another method of detection involves placing a vinegar preparation on the genitals and other affected areas. This turns any warts white, making them easier to see and therefore treat.

For many young women, a Pap smear will show the first presence of a potential HPV infection. A Pap smear is the microscopic examination of cells carefully swabbed from the inside of a woman's vagina or cervix.

Developed by the Greek scientist George Papanicolaou while working at the Woman's Hospital in New York, the Pap smear has helped detect cancerous cells since the early 1940s. This quick, simple, and painless test is credited with dramatically reducing deaths due to cervical cancer.

When the results of a regular Pap smear screening are "positive" or abnormal, your doctor will examine the cervix further, determining if the HPV infection is present. An abnormal Pap smear result could also indicate other conditions that could lead to cancer.

Any abnormal results of a Pap smear screening could result in your doctor wanting to perform another smear for comparison or a test called a biopsy. A biopsy is the removal of a very small piece of tissue from inside the body. After the tissue is removed, it is tested further for any other abnormalities, such as specific strains of the HPV infection. Some of these strains, especially those that show no visible genital

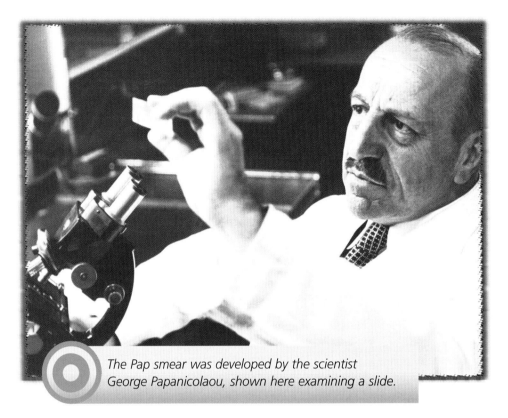

The Pap smear was developed by the scientist George Papanicolaou, shown here examining a slide.

warts, such as strains 16, 18, 31, 33, and 45, are now known to frequently cause cancer.

If genital warts are diagnosed, your doctor will discuss treatment options. The treatment he or she recommends will depend on several factors, including the size, sites, and number of warts to be treated. There are a number of treatment options available, which will be discussed in the next chapter.

What to Do If You Are Pregnant

Tell the doctor or nurse if you are pregnant and seeking treatment for genital warts. He or she can help you select a treatment that won't hurt you or your baby.

According to the ASHA, women with genital warts generally have normal pregnancies and births. While genital warts can be transmitted from mother to baby during the birthing process, this doesn't happen often and can be managed and treated if it occurs.

When you are pregnant, your body and hormones (the chemicals that regulate many of the body's functions) go through many changes. If you have genital warts, they may grow larger as a result of this increase in hormonal activity. You may develop more of them than you would if you were not pregnant. If you have had genital warts in the past, and have been treated prior to becoming pregnant, it is unusual for them to return during your pregnancy.

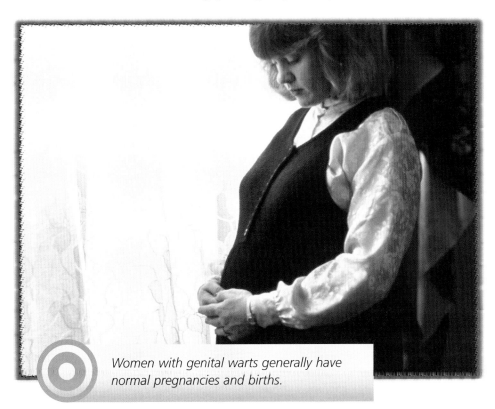

Women with genital warts generally have normal pregnancies and births.

Chapter 3

Treatment and Prevention

HPV is quickly and easily passed from partner to partner through sexual contact. And the sex organs are likely to be the first areas in which any symptoms appear; others are the mouth, throat, and anus.

HPV and Other STDs

It is important to know that if you have been infected with any other STD, such as chlamydia, hepatitis B or C, genital herpes, HIV/AIDS, gonorrhea, and/or syphilis, it is easier for strains of HPV to invade your body. The reason for this is because the body's immune system may not be able to combat more than one infection.

Once HPV has infected the body, it will remain in the cells for an indefinite time, most often in an invisible or latent stage. Still, latent HPV is able to produce symptoms whenever the body's immune system is slowed or compromised. Many situations could cause a recurrence of latent HPV, such as:

◎ **Use of certain medications**

◎ **HIV infection**

◎ **Temporary trauma**

◎ **Serious illnesses**

◎ **Surgery**

◎ **Excessive stress**

Condoms Offer Only Limited Protection

Also known as rubbers, condoms offer protection against the spread of STDs. They also help prevent unplanned pregnancies. To do both effectively, condoms must be used every time a couple has sex. They must also be worn correctly. Widely available, condoms are inexpensive. They can be purchased or obtained at grocery, drug, and convenience stores, STD and health clinics, some public rest rooms, and Planned Parenthood branches.

Condoms offer only limited protection from HPV. This is because condoms cannot cover pubic skin, a

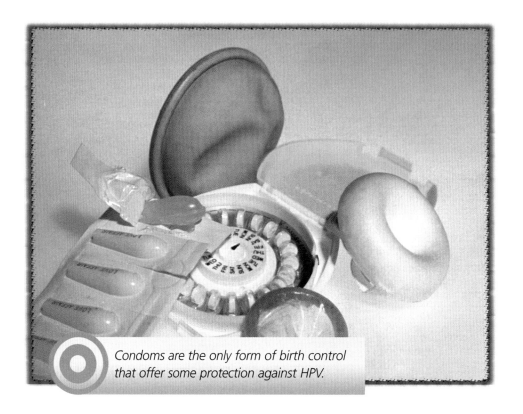

Condoms are the only form of birth control that offer some protection against HPV.

frequent site for genital warts. The only way to completely avoid HPV is to not have sex. Even spermicides like Nonoxynol-9 are noneffective for reducing the spread of HPV. If you notice any broken skin, unusual bumps, sores, or raised areas on you or your partner, don't have sex until a doctor determines the cause.

Latex: Your Best Bet

There are two types of condoms. One is made from latex; the other from animal skin. Only latex condoms protect you against STDs. Condoms made from animal skin do not. This is because viruses and bacteria can easily pass through animal tissue.

The Female Condom

A relatively new and highly effective barrier against pregnancy and sexually transmitted diseases, the female condom is a plastic pouch with rings at each end that hold it in place comfortably. The outer ring remains outside the vagina, partly covering the labia, while the inner ring fits snugly inside. The female condom can be inserted up to several hours before a woman has sex. It must be changed after each sexual encounter.

Oral Sex

Many people think oral sex (mouth to penis or mouth to clitoris or vulva) is safer than intercourse (penis to vagina) when it comes to the spread of STDs. This is not true. STDs can be spread easily during oral sex, although male condoms provide a shield from STD transmission. Another important barrier is a dental dam. A small latex square, the dental dam is placed over the clitoris, vaginal opening, and labia to prevent any exchange of bodily fluids during oral sex.

Abstinence Is Not a Dirty Word

Although most teens would like to believe that nothing unexpected will happen when they have sex, the truth is that you and your partner take risks by becoming sexually active.

You may put pressure on yourself to have sex because you think that all of your peers are "doing it." Believe it or not, many teens are choosing to abstain from—not engage in—sexual activity until they're older. This takes the pressure off sexual activity and allows time to set limits.

There are many good reasons to wait. The younger a teen is when he or she becomes sexually active, the more likely he or she is to catch an STD if exposure occurs. This is because the body hasn't yet stopped growing. You can still show affection and respect for each other by spending time talking, hugging, kissing, holding hands, and sharing common interests in sports, music, or other favorite activities.

Regular Checkups and Pap Smears Are Important

Now that you know how easy it can be to get and spread HPV, you also know how important it is to get checked regularly. If you develop HPV, your risk of developing cancer of the cervix, anus, or penis can increase. All sexually active teens and women should have yearly physicals, including screenings for sexually transmitted diseases. If you have an abnormal Pap smear, be sure to repeat the test as often as your doctor advises. If Pap smears are done annually, the chances are good that any cancer can be completely prevented or caught early, saving your life.

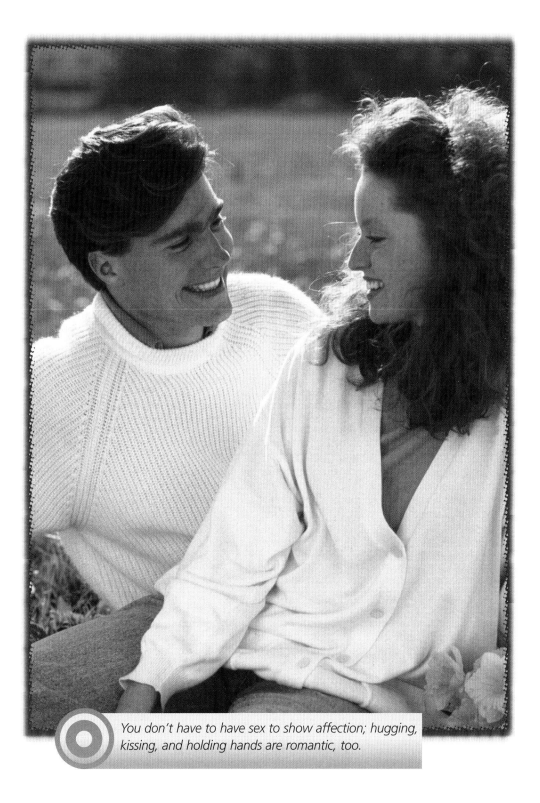

You don't have to have sex to show affection; hugging, kissing, and holding hands are romantic, too.

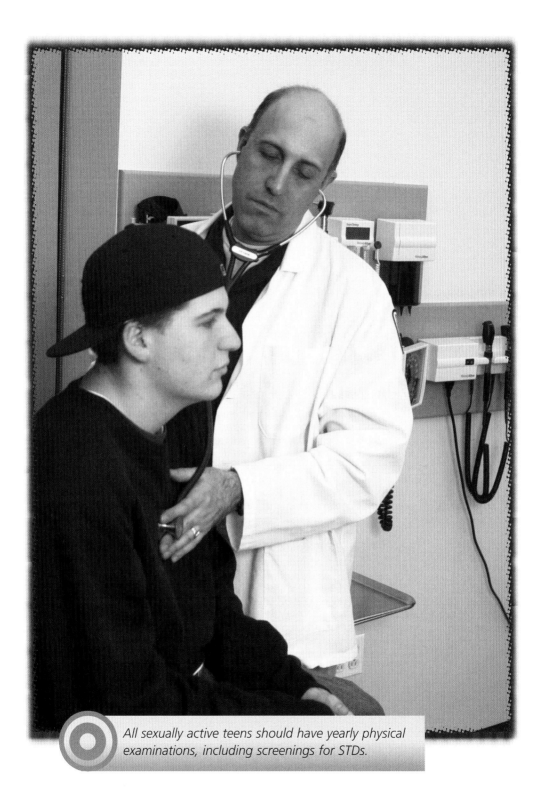

All sexually active teens should have yearly physical examinations, including screenings for STDs.

Despite the Pap smear's effectiveness, women still develop and die from cervical cancer. Elderly and low-income women often lack access to affordable screenings. Younger women may not realize the importance of regular testing. Sometimes, other cultural or social issues keep women from getting the medical care that they need. The bottom line on Pap smears is that all women should have them because they prevent needless deaths.

Treatment Options

Several medications that are used to treat genital warts are available by prescription only and can be easily applied to any external genital warts by the patient. They offer effective relief for any itching, bleeding, or other discomforts warts cause. Medications designed to treat warts on the hands or feet will not work on genital warts and should not be used.

Liquids, Creams, and Gels

◎ **Podofilox: Inexpensive and safe, this medication comes in a liquid or gel that can be applied by the patient to his or her external genital warts. Podofilox should not be used if you are pregnant.**

◎ **Imiquimod cream: Specially designed to treat external genital warts, including those around the anus, this medication is** also safe and easy to apply. Imiquimod stimulates the body's immune system to help fight HPV. This is another cream that should not be used by pregnant women.

Other topical ointments and chemicals must be applied in your doctor's office. These chemicals may cause some pain, burning, and irritation since each destroys the tissue affected by genital warts.

◎ **Podophyllin or Podophyllotoxin: This chemical is derived from a natural plant extract. It must remain on the infected area from one to four hours. Afterward, it is completely washed off and then reapplied weekly for up to six weeks. Extreme care must be taken with podophyllin since it may burn or scar the skin surrounding the genital warts. It isn't recommended if you are pregnant.**

◎ **Trichloroacetic acid or TCA: Another chemical alternative that must be applied to warts in the doctor's office or in a clinic. TCA is a drug that causes genital warts to clot or solidify and is used only to treat small internal or external genital wart clusters.**

TCA is an acceptable treatment for pregnant women.

◉ Fluorouracil: This is a unique chemical that interferes with the DNA synthesis of HPV. Also a topical ointment, Fluorouracil causes a great deal of irritation but is useful in the treatment of vaginal (internal) and vulvar (external) genital warts.

◉ Interferons or IFNs: These drugs are used only after other methods of wart removal have failed. Interferons are antiviral drugs that are injected directly into the wart, sometimes as often as three times per week. IFNs may cause many side effects; other treatments eliminate warts as well or better.

Physical Methods of Wart Removal

Although some of the following wart removal therapies may be painful, your doctor will perform them if other remedies fail. All methods described in this section require anesthesia.

◉ Cryotherapy: This "freezing" method involves the removal of genital warts using liquid nitrogen. This method

destroys warts and the immediate surrounding area. Cryotherapy normally
takes several visits to your doctor over
the course of many weeks and is a safe
method to choose if pregnant.

◎ Laser surgery or therapy: A high-intensity
light is used to remove warts from the
genitals or other areas of the body.
This removal method is effective for
sparing other healthy surrounding
tissue and is safe for pregnant women.
Only specially trained doctors can
perform laser procedures.

◎ Electrosurgery: This method involves
the use of high-frequency currents to
destroy interior tissue affected by
genital warts. This may be an
effective treatment option for internal
cervical venereal warts. Usually,
electrosurgery is even more effective
for eliminating venereal warts than
laser or cryotherapy.

◎ Surgical excision: Surgery is sometimes
preferred over other methods simply
because it tends to cause less overall
pain and allows for improved healing.

Surgical removal of internal venereal warts is a choice made by doctors when warts are extensive.

There Is No Cure for HPV

The treatments described here only get rid of the symptoms; they do not cure HPV or genital warts. Following any treatment, HPV remains in the body. Symptoms can reappear, especially during the first year or so after diagnosis. In many cases, the body's immune system fights HPV so that it causes no further symptoms.

Other Important Considerations

You may be told not to have sex until the treated areas have completely healed. Your partner also should be treated, even if he or she has no symptoms. Do not share or swap medications with your partner.

Be Sure to Ask About:

- The advantage and cost of each treatment your doctor recommends

- Any possible side effects of medication

- What you'll need to do if any itching, bleeding, or pain occurs following treatment

- Whether you'll need more than one treatment

- Precautions you should take if you are pregnant

- When you'll return for any additional treatment or follow-up visits

- Any other questions or concerns that come to mind

Chapter 4

HPV and Cervical Cancer: A Growing Concern

While only a small number of women with an HPV infection will develop cervical cancer, medical researchers now know that particular strains of HPV, such as 16, 18, 31, 33, and 45, are responsible for approximately 99 percent of all cervical cancers.

Cervical cancer is still considered a public health threat. The number of cervical cancer cases diagnosed yearly in the United States is 14,500; of these, 4,800 end in death. Many or all of these deaths are preventable. With early diagnosis and treatment of cervical cell changes, women's lives can be saved.

Researchers think that most of these cervical cancers develop when viruses harm the genes (the body's blueprint for growth and function) that tell the body to produce the right number of normal cells. Because of the virus, the body produces too many abnormal cells.

While cervical cancer can take years to develop, doctors in the United States and Canada are seeing cases in which precancerous cervical changes occur much more quickly.

How the body reacts to HPV depends on many things: the particular strains in a person's body, the ability of the immune system to fight off HPV, and whether or not the person has other risk factors that can make it easier to contract HPV or develop cervical cancer.

This chapter will discuss the cervix, how changes in the cells of the cervix are found, and how to interpret those results. You'll learn about HPV risk factors and how to reduce your risk of HPV infection. You'll also learn about a test that checks for the presence of HPV in women and can isolate strains of HPV in the body.

More About the Cervix

The cervix is at the lower end of the uterus and connects the uterus with the vagina. The cervix and its opening, called the os, allow the blood lost during menstruation to pass from the uterus, into the vagina, and out of the body. If you have a baby, the os will expand to allow the baby to travel from the uterus to the vagina during birth.

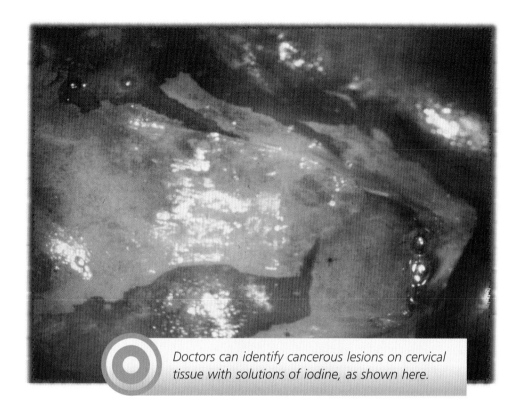

Doctors can identify cancerous lesions on cervical tissue with solutions of iodine, as shown here.

Growing teenage girls need to understand yet another important fact about the cervix. Because the body continues to grow until the age of twenty-one, the cervix is not fully developed. This fact makes young women more likely to become infected with HPV if they have sex with an infected partner.

The "transformation zone"—the area found between the vagina and the cervix—is lower in the bodies of young girls and teenagers than it is in adult women. As young women grow into adulthood, the cervix and uterus develop more fully, gradually shifting higher into the body. Until this growth is completed, girls are more vulnerable to HPV infection and other STDs. If a girl has sex with an infected partner before the age of twenty-one, her partner's penis can reach beyond the vagina and into the body's immature cervix, therefore increasing the risk of infection.

While the subject of HPV and cervical cancer may be frightening, there are many simple steps you can take to minimize your risk if you are a girl:

◎ **Put off sex until the age of twenty-one or after. Waiting cuts your chances of developing cervical cancer dramatically. It also allows your cervix to fully develop. Women who have sex before the age of sixteen are at greater risk for cervical cancer.**

◎ **Limit the number of people you have sex with. If your partner has had sex with many people, your risk of HPV infection increases. Choose someone who has had fewer partners and is willing to have sex only with you.**

◎ **Demand that your partner always use a condom every time you have sex. This limits your exposure to other STDs and decreases potential stress on the body's immune system.**

◎ Avoid sex with high-risk partners. A high-risk partner is someone who has had many partners, has a history of STD infection or partners with that history, or began having sex earlier than age sixteen.

◎ Follow your doctor's advice about how often Pap smears should be done. (The American Cancer Society recommends yearly Pap smears and pelvic exams for all sexually active females and any woman over the age of eighteen.) Be especially alert for any symptoms of genital warts, vaginal discharge, or changes in your period.

◎ Avoid smoking. Research suggests that because smoking stresses the body's immune system, it makes it easier to become infected with HPV.

◎ Avoid consumption of alcohol. Research has proven that there is a definitive connection between cervical cancer and high levels of alcohol consumption.

◎ Maintain a level of wellness. Low levels of vitamin A, vitamin C, folic acid, and beta-carotene could contribute to the development of cervical cancer. Adhering to a healthy diet and proper hydration, combined with other healthy life choices, helps keep your immune system in shape, too. A healthy immune system is your best defense against HPV or any STD infection.

What Happens During a Pap Smear?

If you are a young woman, during a visit to your doctor or clinic, you will first undergo a pelvic exam. The doctor will examine the inside of your vagina, uterus, and ovaries for any swelling, bumps, or other changes. This takes only a few minutes.

The doctor then takes a Pap smear, a small swab of cells from the surface of your cervix. The surface of your cervix is made up of layers of cells, called the epithelium. Epithelial cells are either flat (squamous) or long and thin (columnar). The doctor places this cellular material on a slide and sends it out to a pathology lab for examination. The slide is checked to see if these squamous or columnar cervical cells are normal or if there are any changes that could, if undiagnosed and untreated, later develop into cancer.

If the cells don't appear normal, the Pap smear will be repeated. If the results of the second smear are normal, your doctor may ask you to have another test

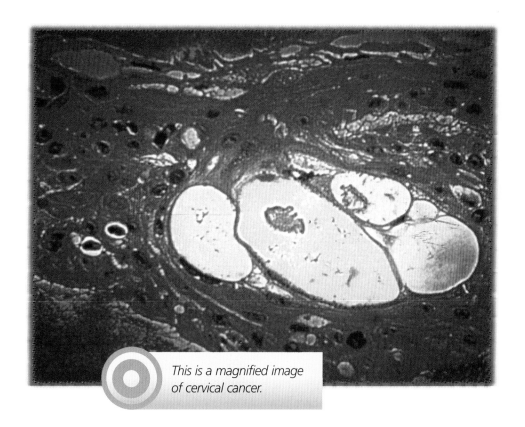

This is a magnified image of cervical cancer.

in a few months. If the second smear is abnormal, however, other specialized tests may be done.

Pap smears are screening tests that are intended to show changes in the surface cells and tissue of the cervix. Not all cell changes signal cancer, so don't panic if your doctor tells you your Pap smear shows changes in your cervix.

Colposcopy

When doctors want a better look at the tissue in your cervix following an abnormal Pap smear, they may use a special magnifying lens with a light attached to

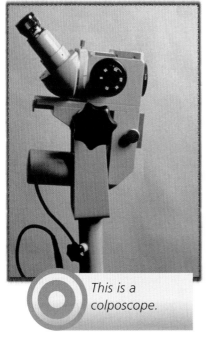

This is a colposcope.

it, called a colposcope. During the examination, certain staining liquids, such as acetic acid or Lougal's iodine, are applied to the cervix to identify cancerous lesions. The colposcopy procedure can help identify changes in cervical cells, abnormal groups of cells on the cervix, or the development of cancer. In many circumstances, depending on the results of the colposcopy test, your doctor may then suggest that you undergo a test called a biopsy.

Biopsy

If a closer exam is needed to see these cellular changes, your doctor may request a biopsy. During a biopsy, a small bit of cervical tissue (cells from the inside of the cervix) is removed and examined in a pathology lab. This test takes less than fifteen minutes and is practically painless (some patients experience slight cramping or bleeding afterward). A biopsy test allows your doctor the ability to analyze the exact cells that are causing abnormalities in the Pap smear results. These results tell your doctor more about the cell changes he or she has found in your cervix.

Hybrid Capture II HPV Test

Doctors now have a test they can use to confirm HPV infection in women. Called the Hybrid Capture II HPV test, it is intended to help doctors locate which strains of HPV a woman has in her body. The HPV test is used after repeated Pap smears have shown cervical cell abnormalities. It can help identify a woman's chances of developing cervical cancer. This allows doctors to watch the situation carefully and treat cervical changes before any cancer develops.

A positive HPV test does not mean that you have cervical cancer. It simply means that you've been infected with HPV. Most women with HPV don't develop cancer, but knowing and understanding your risk can help you make better decisions about your health.

Dysplasia

Dysplasia is the medical word that describes changes in the cells of a woman's cervix. These changes happen before any cancer appears and include variations in the shapes of the cells on the surface of the cervix. Doctors classify dysplasia as mild, moderate, or severe, depending on the abnormality seen when the cells are examined.

Dysplasia does not necessarily develop into cervical cancer; your doctor may suggest monitoring the cell changes closely with more frequent testing, or he or she may treat the condition if it is moderate or severe. If your dysplasia is mild, it may go away on its own.

Many women with dysplasia never have any symptoms or discomfort, but any changes in your period, abdominal pain, or discharge from your vagina should be reported to your doctor immediately.

Heavy bleeding, longer than normal periods, bleeding after sex, vaginal discharge that smells, fatigue, and pain are some of the symptoms signaling cervical cancer. They may not appear until the later stages of the disease and should never be ignored.

Many teens feel nervous or anxious about pelvic exams, Pap smears, and the many other tests doctors may perform. You may be concerned about discomfort and have questions about your body, what the results may mean, and what you'll need to do to take care of yourself. This is normal. If you have questions, ask your doctor or nurse for more information.

Chapter 5

Penile and Anal Cancers

In addition to causing cervical and other cancers in women, certain high-risk strains of HPV (strains 16, 18, 31, 33, and 45) can also lead to cancer of the penis or anus in men. According to the American Cancer Society, approximately 1,100 men will be newly diagnosed with cancer of the penis this year; 300 deaths will result from penile cancer in the same period.

Anal cancers that affect both men and women are rare but appear to be increasing. Of the 3,400 newly diagnosed cases predicted for this year, about 1,400 will occur in men. Two hundred men are expected to die from anal cancer in that time.

Although these cancers are uncommon, understanding their connection to HPV, as well as to other known risk factors, can help you make important decisions about your sexual habits and health.

Penile Cells and Cancer

Each part of the penis is made up of various kinds of cells that form the skin, nerves, muscle, and the three small chambers that contain an extensive web of blood vessels and tissue. A different type of cancer could invade each of these groups. This is significant because where a particular cancer grows helps doctors know how it can impact a man's health, how quickly it is likely to spread, and the best methods for treating it.

Most cancers of the penis—about 95 percent—result from flat, scaly skin cells known as squamous cells. Squamous cell cancers can find a home anywhere on the penis, but they usually settle on either the glans (the tip of the penis) or the foreskin (the retractable covering that hoods the glans) unless a man has been circumcised (had his foreskin surgically removed). These cancers generally develop quite slowly and are curable if found early.

Adenocarcinoma of the penis is a rare type of squamous cell cancer that advances from the sweat glands found in penile skin. When adenocarcinoma occurs in the skin of a man's penis, it is called Paget's disease. These cancer cells initially spread in the skin. At later stages, these cells develop in the lymph nodes (tiny groups of disease-fighting cells that are part of your body's immune system).

Another infrequent kind of squamous cell cancer occurs in both men and women. Often called

Bushke-Lowenstein tumor, this cancer can be found on the genitals of men and women as well as on the skin, or inside the anus, mouth, or larynx. It closely resembles noncancerous genital warts and rarely spreads to other parts of the body.

Other penile cancers can form from the cells that manufacture your skin's color or pigment. Known as melanomas, these cancers normally appear on skin that has been repeatedly exposed to sunlight or sunburn. Melanomas may also develop on the penis or in other less exposed areas and are responsible only for about 2 percent of penile cancers. Although this is a very small number, melanomas can grow and spread very quickly, making them an aggressive, and sometimes deadly, form of cancer.

Sarcomas are cancers that evolve from penile muscle cells, blood vessel cells, or the cells of other membranes of the penis. They constitute about 1 percent of all cancers of the penis. Basal cell cancers also normally grow on sun-exposed portions of the body. Unlike melanomas, these cancers develop slowly and do not often spread to other areas. They account for less than 2 percent of penile cancers. A factor that greatly influences the onset and outcome of treatment is waiting too long. The earlier and more quickly you respond by getting medical attention, the greater your chances of staying healthy. See your doctor at the first signs of any abnormality.

Squamous Cell Cancers and Dysplasia

Squamous cancers usually develop after precancerous changes in the cells of penile tissue occur. Referred to by doctors as dysplasia or penile intraepithelial neoplasia, these precancerous changes happen slowly and involve only cells on the top layer of the penile skin.

A man with precancerous dysplasia may develop one or many warts, which can range from being virtually invisible to appearing like a miniature head of cauliflower. Other unusual growths or irritated sections of skin can also indicate dysplasia. These changes most often occur on the glans or foreskin but may also happen along the shaft of the penis. It is important to remember that although many types of warts are benign (not cancerous), any change in the appearance of the penis should be immediately examined by a doctor.

A Wide Array of Symptoms

Symptoms of penile cancer vary. They include painless ulcers on the glans, foreskin, or shaft. A reddish, velvety rash on the penis, sores, blisters, crusty or patchy white areas, a thickening of the skin, an enduring, smelly discharge from under the foreskin, or bleeding, as well as swollen lymph nodes in and around the groin, can also signal cancer. Swelling at the end of the penis or in the groin is an additional signal that should not be ignored. Symptoms that develop beneath the foreskin may be difficult to see until it is retracted. In some instances, a man may have no symptoms until the cancer has advanced to later stages.

Diagnosing Penile Cancers

The first step in detecting any cancer involves a thorough inspection of the penis by a doctor. When abnormalities are found, a biopsy is done to confirm the presence and type of cancer. The biopsied tissue is carefully checked in a pathology lab. This removed tissue can also reveal at which stage the cancer has been found and what future tests need to be conducted.

Seeing Is Believing

The doctor may perform an ultrasound, a computed tomography scan or CT scan, or a magnetic resonance imaging test or MRI. Each of these allow the doctor to see the cancer quickly, painlessly, and fully, with virtually no discomfort to the patient. All of these tests provide doctors with additional information they must have to effectively treat any cancer. The treatment a patient receives depends on the type of cancer, its stage of development, and its location, as well as other factors.

◎ **Ultrasound: This is a test in which sound waves are used to explore and provide images of tissue using a special probe and a computer. With this information,** the doctor can determine how deeply cancer has spread into a man's penis.

◉ Magnetic resonance imaging or MRI: This test uses magnetic fields to examine and fully picture cancer and the areas surrounding it. An MRI can display soft tissues clearly.

◉ Computed tomography or CT scan: This test can offer doctors yet another method for viewing the body's organs from many different angles. To emphasize a particular area, they may inject patients with a dye. This harmless solution allows doctors to better define the tissue under study.

Risk Factors for Penile Cancer Include:

◉ HPV infection: This disease is seen as a preventable risk factor for penile and anal cancer. Currently, there is no test a man can take to detect HPV infection, such as the Hybrid Capture II HPV test for women. Young men can reduce the risk by having sex later, reducing the number of sex partners, using condoms to practice safe sex, not smoking, reducing stress on the immune system by not contracting other STDs, eating healthily, and getting adequate exercise and rest. Also, keeping the area under the fore-skin clean and free of infection is another suggestion. (Avoid smegma, an oily, sometimes cheeselike substance that can build up under the foreskin if the man is not careful about keeping that area clean.)

◎ Smoking: Believed to alter the DNA of penile cells and contribute to the development of cancerous cells, researchers have noticed a correlation between cancer development and smoking, especially in males who also have HPV in their bodies.

◎ Phimosis: A condition in which the foreskin becomes hard to pull back. Phimosis may lead to too much smegma around the tip of the penis, making it harder to keep clean and raising possible cancer risks.

◎ Psoriasis, drug, and light interaction: According to information provided by the American Cancer Society, men with the skin condition known as psoriasis who are treated with ultraviolet light

and/or a drug called Psorafen tend to have higher levels of penile cancer.

Anal Cancer

The "butt" of endless jokes and giggles, the anus is actually part of an intricate system designed to rid the body of waste. It is found at the lowest end of your large intestine. Known as the rectum, this portion of the intestine serves as the collection point for waste (feces) that passes out of the anal opening. The uppermost part of the large intestine is called the colon.

Anal tissues, like other parts of the body, are composed of many different kinds of cells, including epithelial (outer or surface) squamous cells as well as dendritic cells or melanocytes (those that produce pigment). Several different cancers can grow in these cells. Their locations and types tell doctors how to treat them.

Many different growths can develop in the anal epithelium. Some are not cancerous, or benign. Others begin harmlessly enough but become cancerous as cells change form. As discussed in previous chapters, the term for precancerous cell change is dysplasia.

Most cancers of the anus develop from squamous cells. Called squamous cell carcinomas, these cancers begin on the surface of anal skin. Some spread beyond the surface and attack surrounding tissues. Other anal cancers include adenocarcinomas. These often develop in glands underneath the skin. Glands are cells, groups of cells, or organs of the body that produce and secrete fluids such as mucous or sweat. Basal cell cancers and melanomas can also develop in or on anal tissue, but this is uncommon.

Risk Factors for Anal Cancer Include:

⊚ HPV infection: **HPV can be spread through anal (as well as vaginal or oral) sex. Some of the warts produced by certain strains of HPV can become cancerous.**

⊚ Smoking: **According to the American Cancer Society, if you smoke, you are eight times more likely than a nonsmoker to suffer from cancer of the anus.**

⊚ Reduced immunity: **A compromised immune system increases your chances of developing anal cancer. This includes people with HIV, the virus that causes AIDS, or those who have had organ transplants and need to take medications to prevent organ rejection.**

⊚ Engaging in high-risk sexual activity: **Research suggests that increased high-risk sexual activities such as receptive anal sex could possibly increase a person's chances of developing anal cancer.**

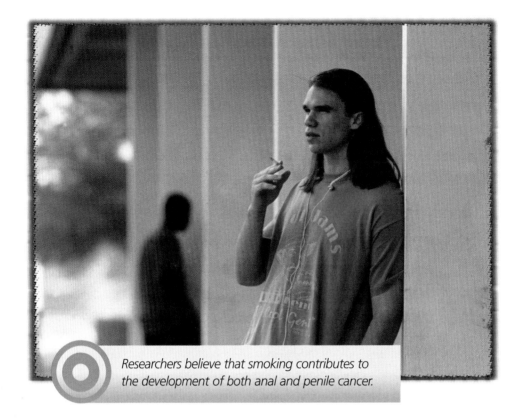

Researchers believe that smoking contributes to the development of both anal and penile cancer.

Symptoms of Anal Cancer:

◎ Pain in your anal area

◎ Anal itching

◎ Straining during bowel movements

◎ A change in the frequency of your bowel movements

◎ Any swelling in the anal or groin areas

◎ Anal discharge

Diagnosing Anal Cancer

Anal cancer is sometimes found following a physical exam or a digital rectal exam in which the doctor feels the inside of the anus and rectum for any signs of abnormality, such as tissue masses, polyps (projection growths), or abscesses (tissues that produce mucus). Similar to the screening tests for cervical cancer in women, a swab is often inserted into the anal canal to collect a cell sample. The sample is then sent to a pathology lab for further examination and testing. Medical staff refers to this test as an anal Pap smear.

If any abnormal growth is detected, your doctor may recommend any of several procedures that allow him or her to view anal tissue. An anoscopy, (similar to a colposcopy where a lighted instrument assists doctors in viewing interior tissues), a biopsy, or an examination of swollen lymph nodes may follow this detection. If cancer is found, tests such as CT scans or ultrasound can help determine its type and stage of development.

Anal cancer is rare and usually curable if found early. It is usually treated with a combination of radiation and chemotherapy—both are treatments to stop cancerous cells from reproducing. As with penile cancer, it is best to understand your risk factors, particularly those connected with the spread of HPV, so you can make healthy decisions.

Glossary

abnormal Pap smear results may be defined as abnormal or positive, meaning that the results have tested positive for a certain amount of inflamed, irritated, or abnormal cells or cellular changes.

abstinence Not having sex or engaging in certain other sexual activities.

active A phase of a disease in which there are symptoms or infectious activity.

anus The bodily opening from the rectum to the outside of the body.

benign Noncancerous.

biopsy The clinical process of removing a tiny tissue sample from inside the body for closer, microscopic examination.

cancer A disease marked by abnormal cell growth. Some cancer types spread deeply into tissues while others remain in one area.

cervix The narrow portion of the uterus that opens into the vagina.

colposcopy A special examination that allows a closer inspection of the cervix. During a colposcopy procedure, a microscope called a colposcope is used to magnify the cervix. This helps the doctor look for visible signs of internal genital warts or an HPV infection.

condom A latex sheath that fits over the penis and helps prevent pregnancy and exposure to sexually transmitted diseases. Female condoms line the inside of a woman's vagina and cover the outer labia.

dysplasia Medical term for cell changes that occur before cancer develops.

genital Referring to the genitals, penis, scrotum, or testes in men, and labia, vagina, or clitoris in women.

genital wart A raised skin growth or bump that develops as a result of HPV infection. Genital warts can be very small and difficult to notice, or large, flat, and raised. They can appear singly or in clusters resembling cauliflower.

hormones Chemicals that regulate the body's growth and many of its functions.

human papillomavirus A group of viruses that can cause warts to develop on or inside the body, particularly in the genital area. Some strains of human papillomavirus also lead to certain types of cancers in men and women. Also called HPV.

inactive A phase of a disease in which there are no symptoms or infectious activity. The infecting organism is present, but dormant.

labia The outer lips or opening to a woman's vagina.

latent HPV A period of inactivity for HPV, during which no symptoms may be apparent. Symptoms may reappear at any time.

Pap smear A procedure used by a doctor to check for abnormal cells in the cervix that could lead to cancer. A small amount of tissue is swabbed from inside the vaginal area and sent to a pathology lab for further examination. Anal Pap smears can also be performed.

penis The external sex organ of a male.

precancerous This term is used to describe cells that may be on the way to becoming cancerous but are not yet truly cancerous.

STD A disease, such as HPV or AIDS, that is transmitted through sexual contact with an infected person.

vagina Passage from a woman's uterus or womb to the outside of the body.

virus An organism that invades and uses the cells of the body to reproduce itself.

Where to Go for Help

In the United States

The American Cancer Society
1599 Clifton Road NE
Atlanta, GA 30329-4251
(800) ACS-2345 (227-2345)
Web site: http://www.cancer.org

The American Social Health Association
(ASHA)
P.O. Box 13827
Research Triangle Park, NC 27713
Web site: http://www.ashastd.org
Confidential brochures on HPV as well as information
on support groups are available from ASHA. It also
runs the National HPV and Cervical Cancer Hotline
that can be contacted between 2 PM and 7 PM EST,
Monday through Friday, at (919) 361-4848. This is part

of the National HPV and Cervical Cancer Prevention Resource Center.

Centers for Disease Control and Prevention (CDC)
National STD Hotline
(800) 227-8922
Web site: http://www.cdc.gov

National Cancer Institute
Public Inquiries Office
Building 31, Room 10A31
31 Center Drive
MSC 2580
Bethesda, MD 20892-2580
(301) 435-3848
(800) 4-CANCER (442-6237)
Web site: http://www.nci.nih.gov

Planned Parenthood Federation of America
810 Seventh Avenue
New York, NY 10019
(212) 541-7800 or (800) 230-PLAN
Web site: http://www.plannedparenthood.org

In Canada

Canadian Cancer Society
National Office

10 Alcorn Avenue, Suite 200
Toronto, ON M4V 3B1
(416) 961-7223
(888) 939-3333
Web site: http://www.cancer.ca

Health Canada
Address Locator 0904A
Ottawa, ON K1A 0K9
(613) 957-2991
Web site: http://www.hc-sc.gc.ca

Planned Parenthood Federation of Canada
1 Nicholas Street, Suite 430
Ottawa, ON K1N 7B7
(613) 241-4474
Web site: http://www.ppfc.ca

Population and Health Branch (formerly the
Laboratory Centre for Disease Control)
Bureau of Infectious Diseases
Health Protection Branch
Health Canada
Tunney's Pasture
Ottawa, ON K1A 0L2
Postal Locator 0603E1
Web site: http://www.hc-sc.gc.ca/hpb/lcdc/index.html

For Further Reading

Byers, Ann. *Sexually Transmitted Diseases: A Hot Issue*. Springfield, NJ: Enslow Publishers, 1999.

Curran, Christine Perdan. *Sexually Transmitted Diseases*. Springfield, NJ: Enslow Publishers, 1998.

Dudley, William, ed. *Sexually Transmitted Diseases*. San Diego, CA: Greenhaven Press, 1999.

McCoy, Kathy, and Charles Wibbelsman. *The Teenage Body Book*. New York: Perigee, 1999.

Moe, Barbara. *Everything You Need to Know About Sexual Abstinence*. New York: The Rosen Publishing Group, Inc., 1996.

Nardo, Don. *Teen Sexuality*. San Diego, CA: Lucent Books, 1997.

Index

About the Author

Elizabeth Carter is a writer currently living in Florida. She shares her home with three fabulous felines and enjoys traveling to places near and far. Her areas of specialization include drug and alcohol abuse, eating disorders, and mental health issues.

Photo Credits

Cover and pp. 21, 24, 41, 42 © Custom Medical; p. 4 © Michael Paras/International Stock; pp. 8, 28 by Antonio Mari; p. 11 © Dr. F.C. Skvara/Peter Arnold, Inc.; p. 18 © Corbis; p. 20 © Corbis/Bettmann; pp. 27, 54 © Pictor; p. 37 © Peter Arnold, Inc.

Design and Layout

Thomas Forget